Food Choices

For all the kind children out there.
Especially Silas & Cedric.

All animals need to eat to keep their bodies healthy and strong

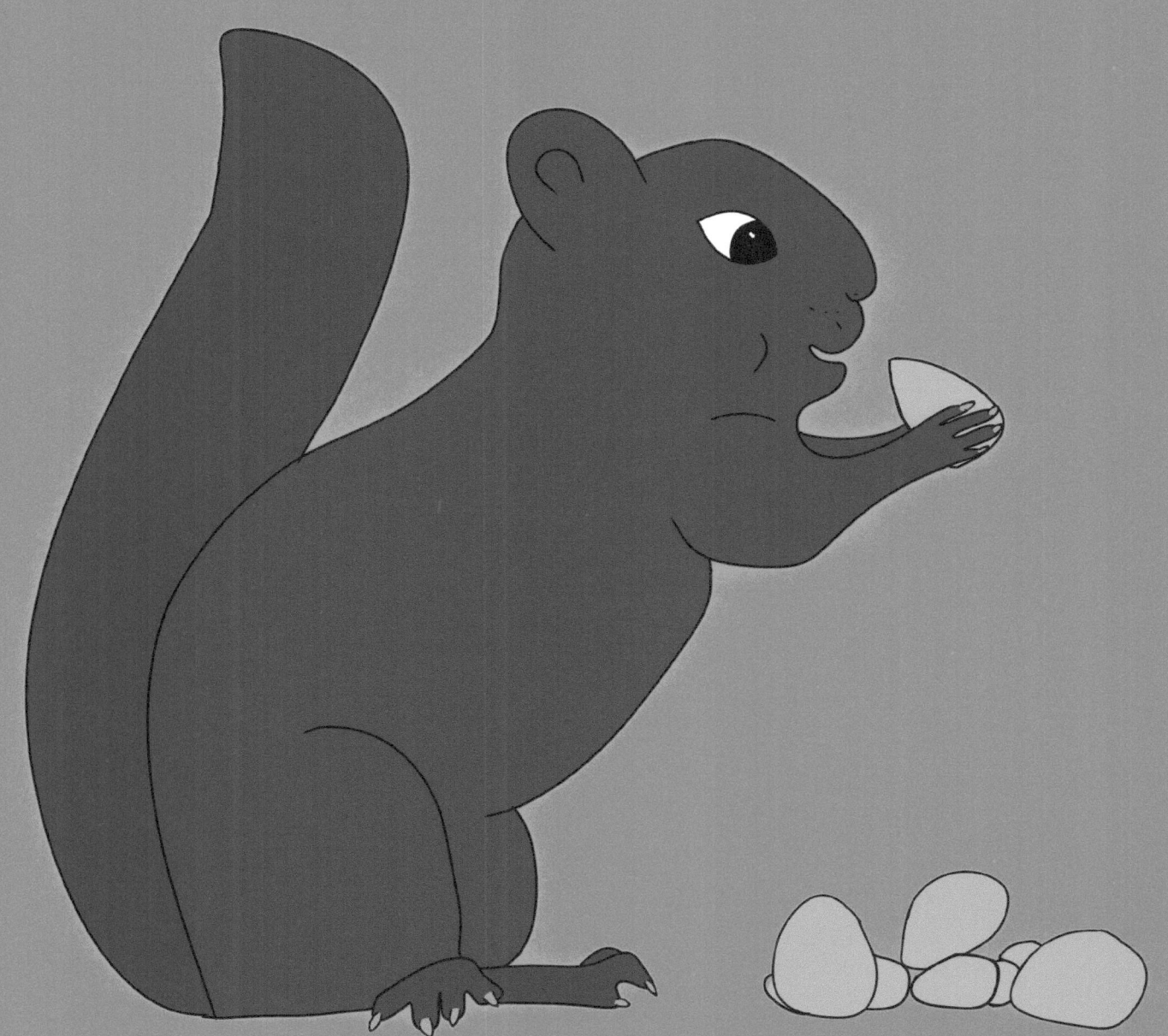

Some animals get their energy from eating plants

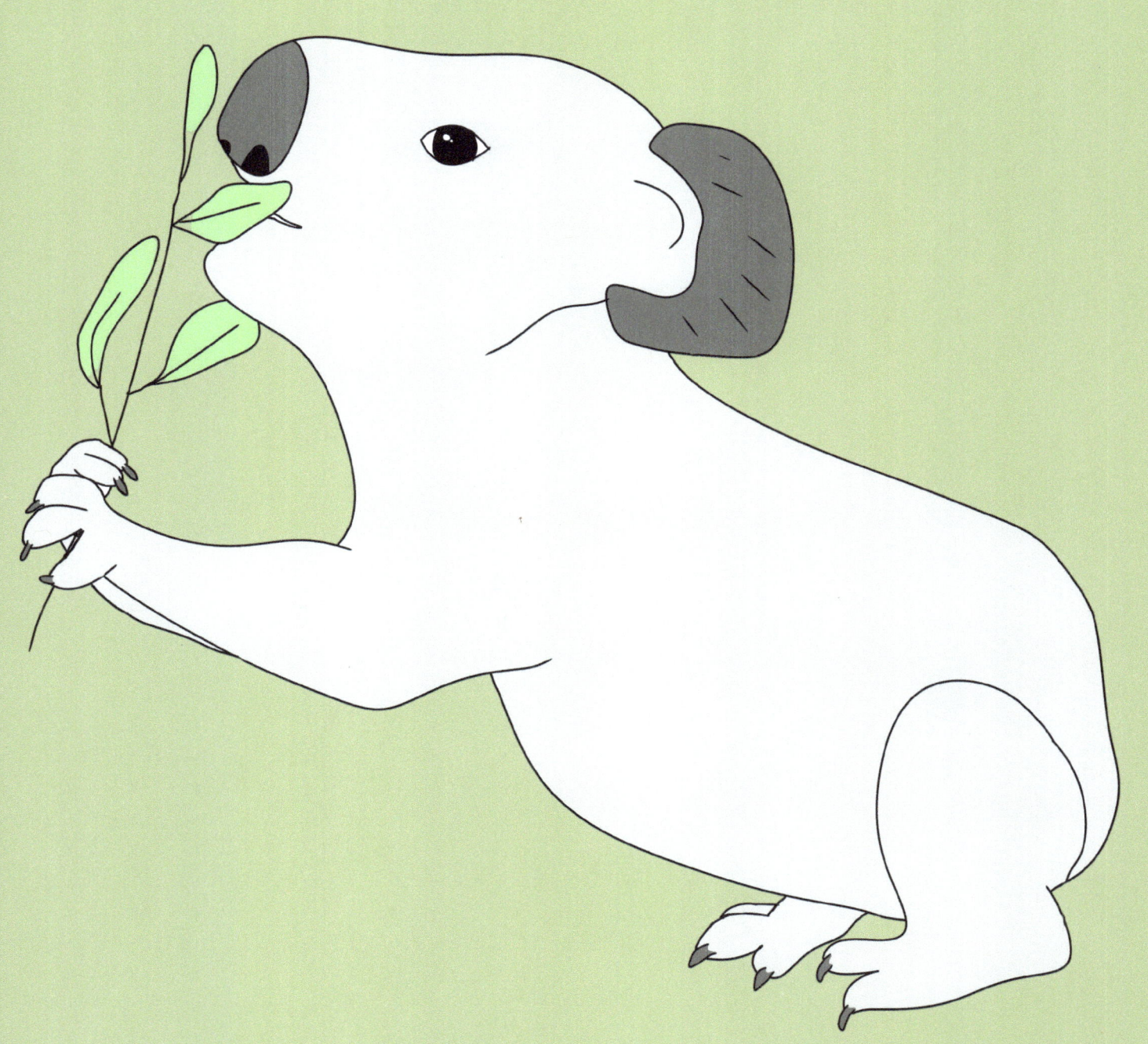

Some animals nourish their bodies by eating other animals

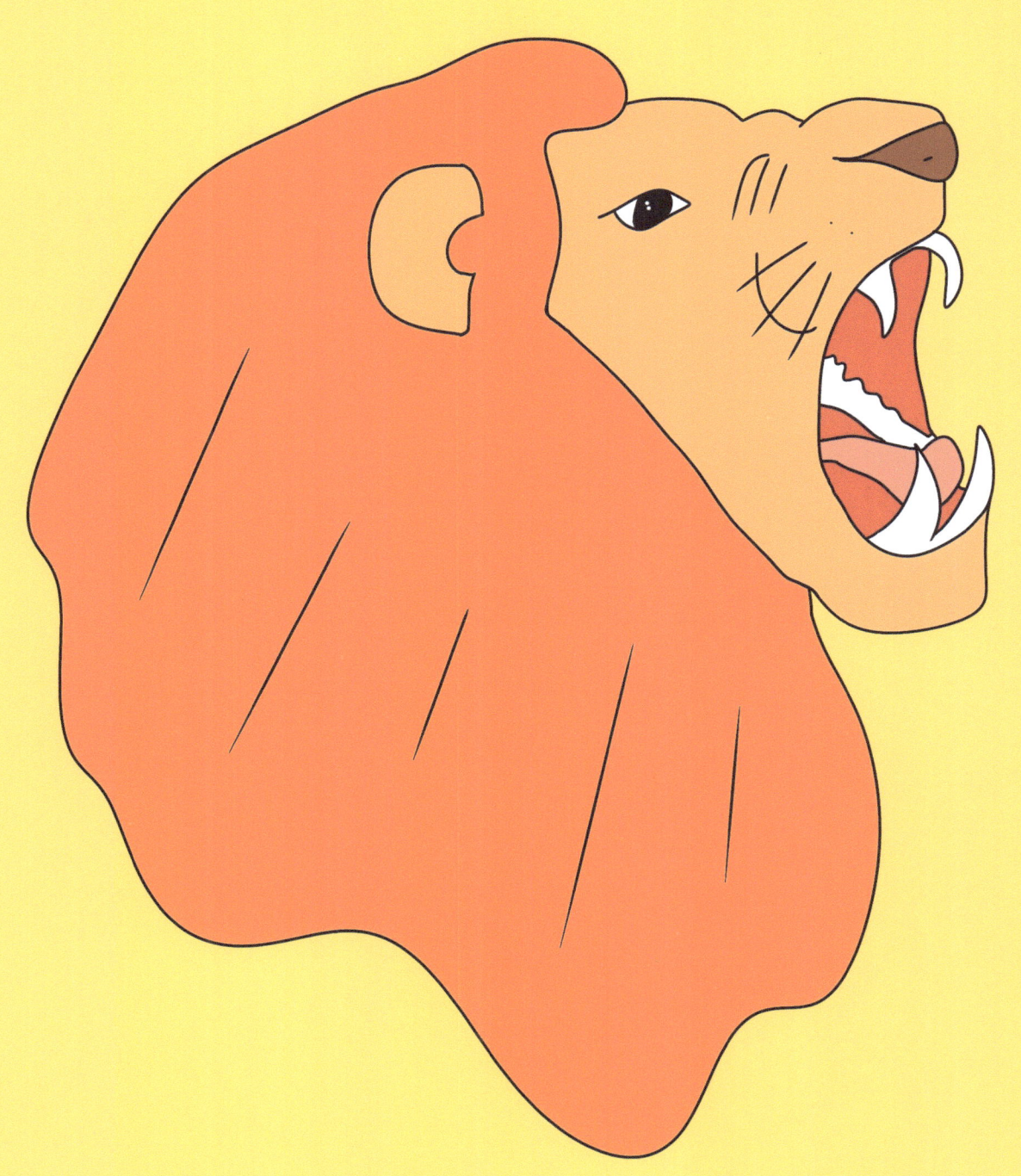

Humans are animals too

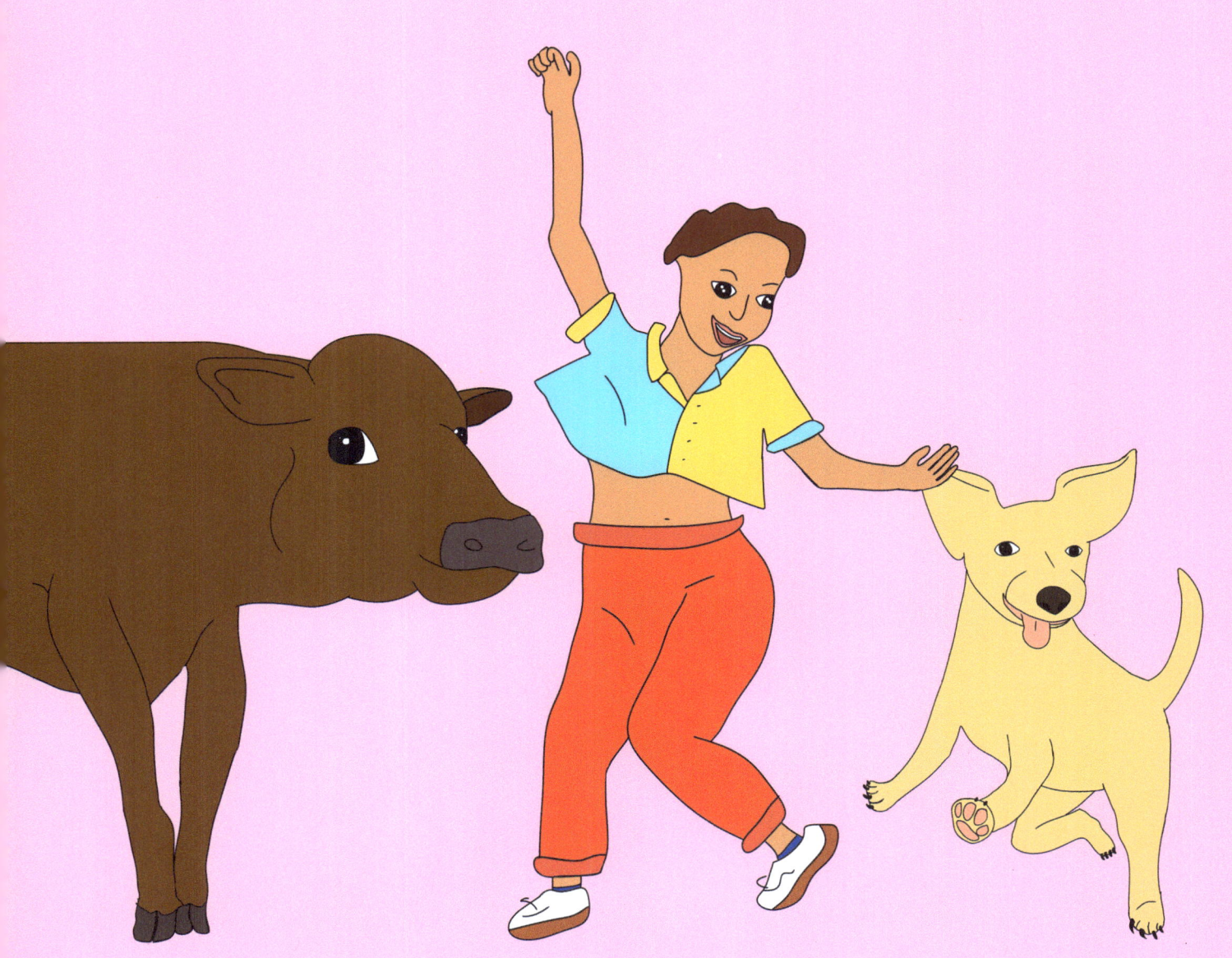

Other animals use their instincts to decide what to eat

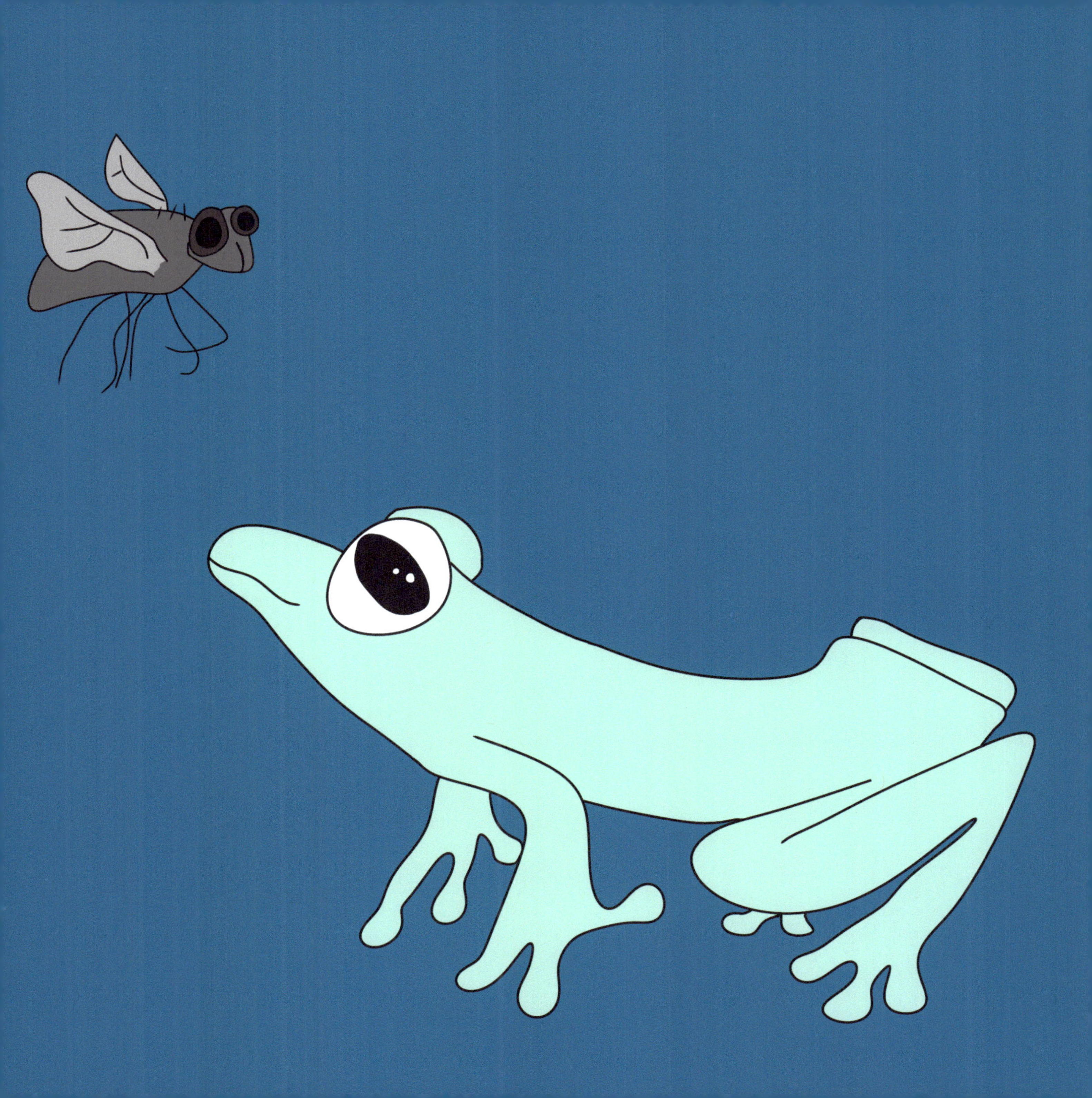

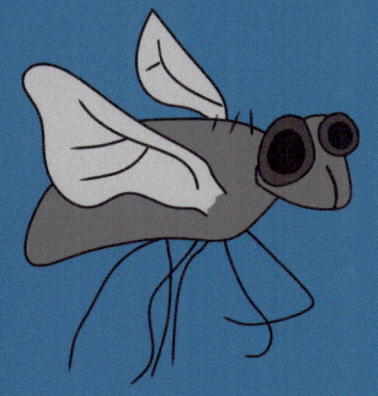

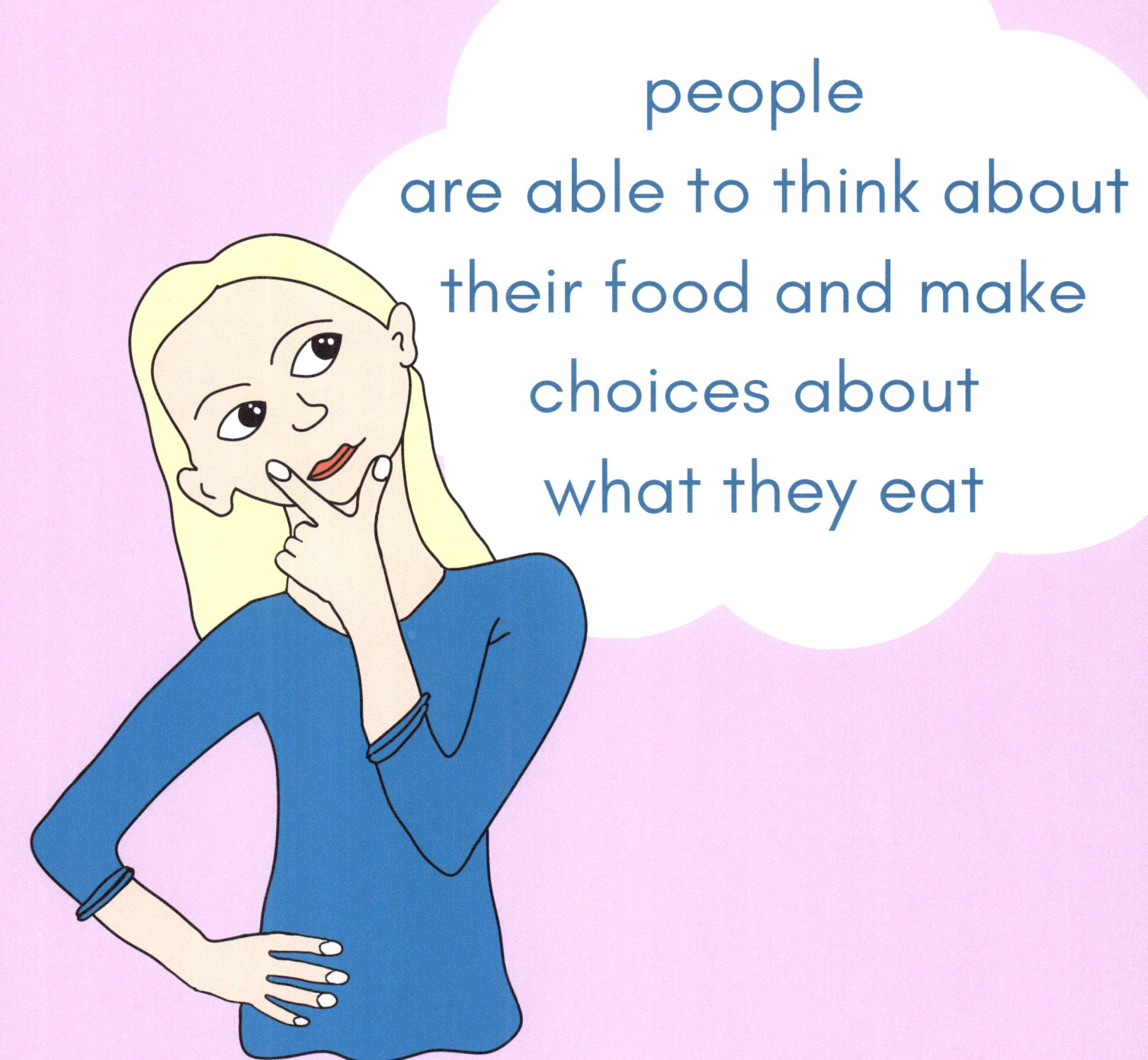

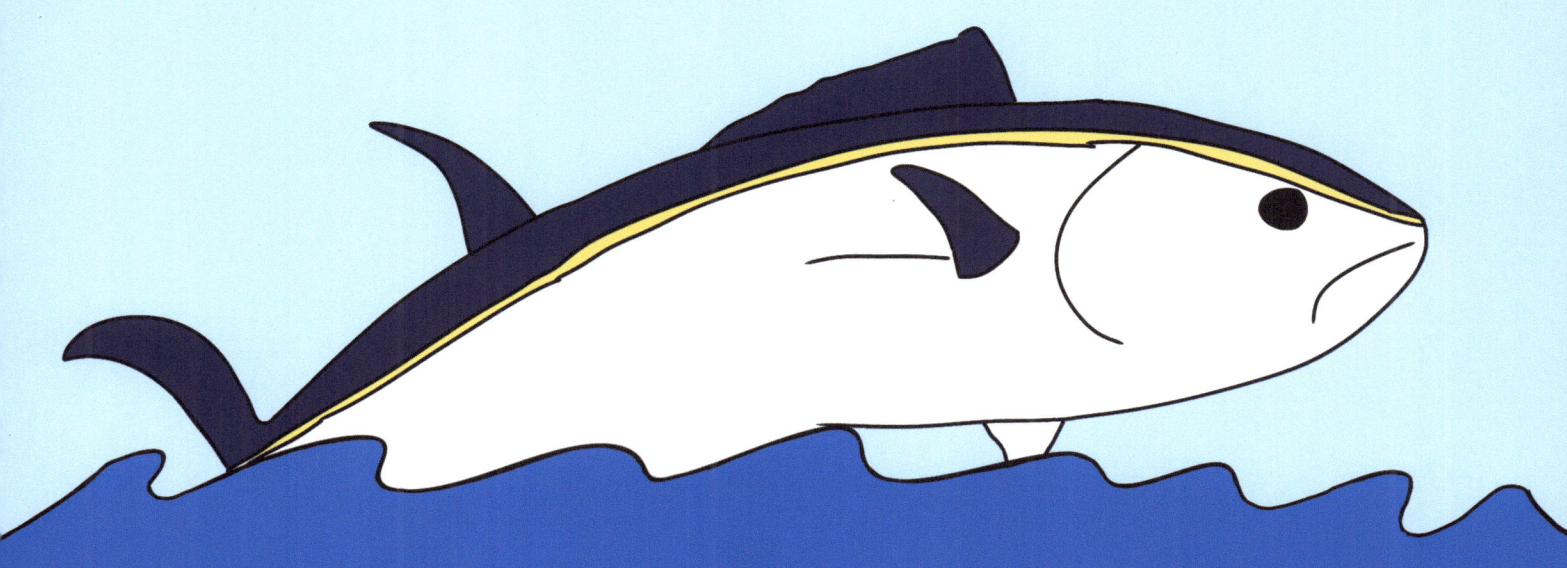

Some people choose to eat other animals as well

People call parts of animal bodies that they eat "meat"

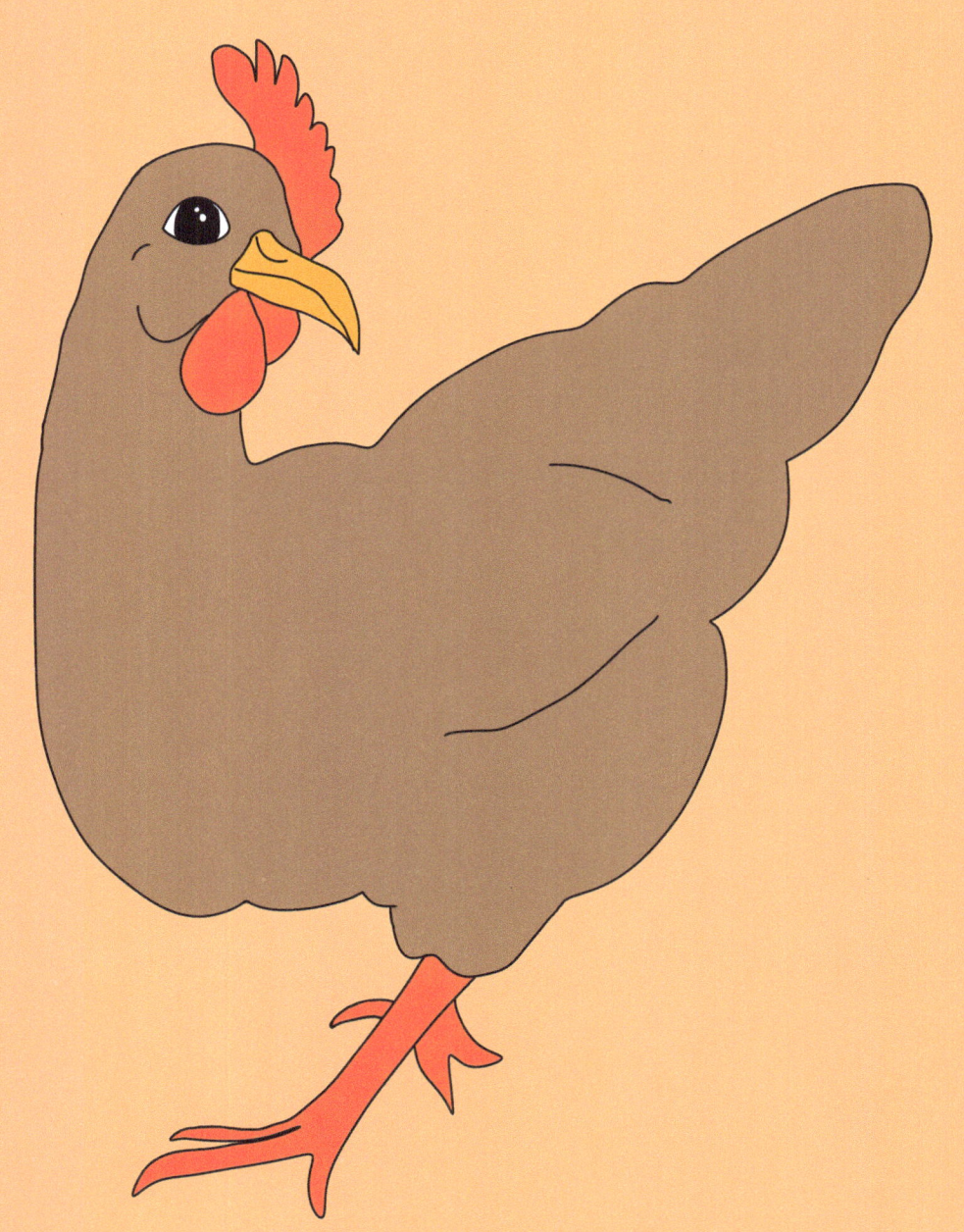

For people to eat meat, animals have to get hurt and die

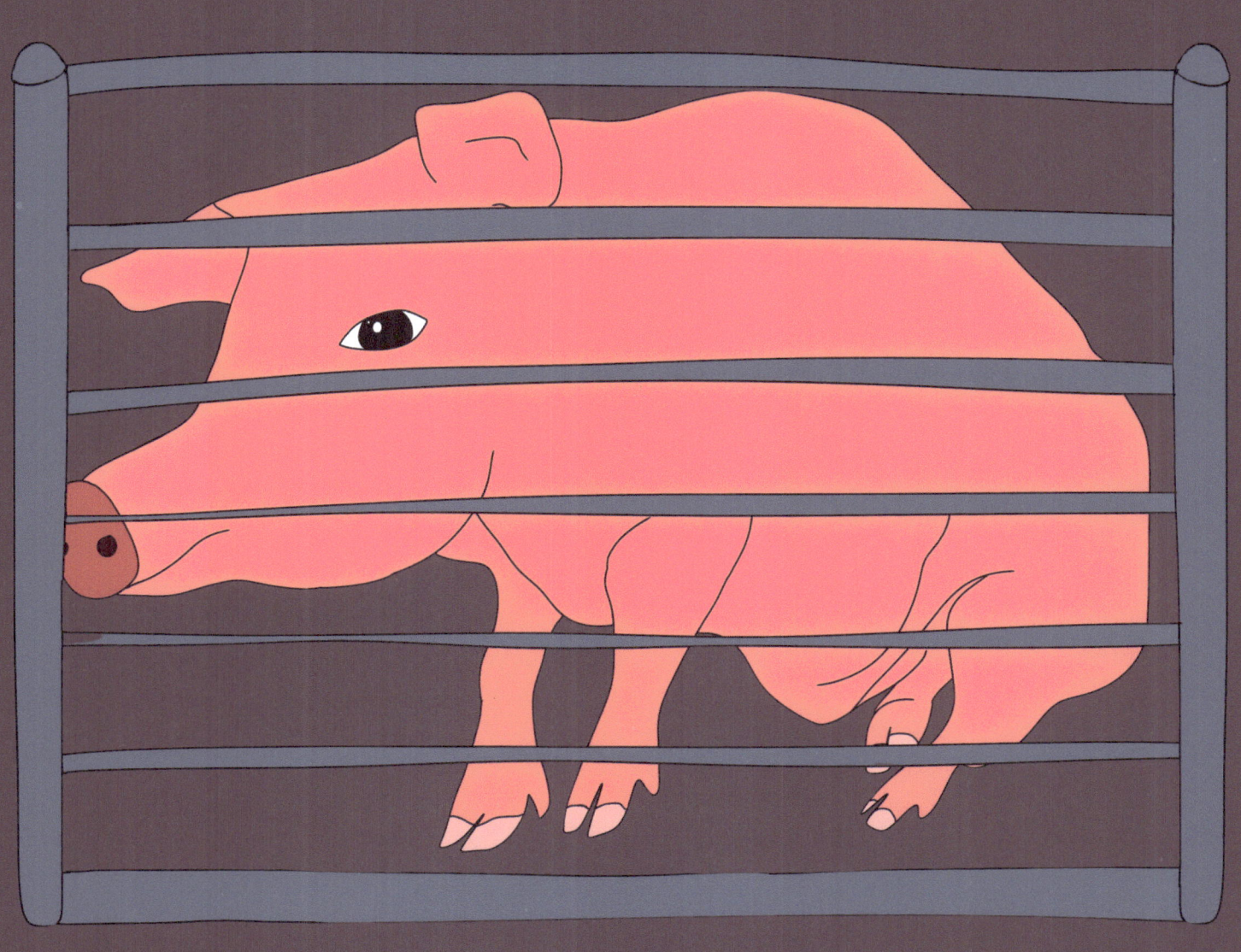

People also choose to eat other things made by animals

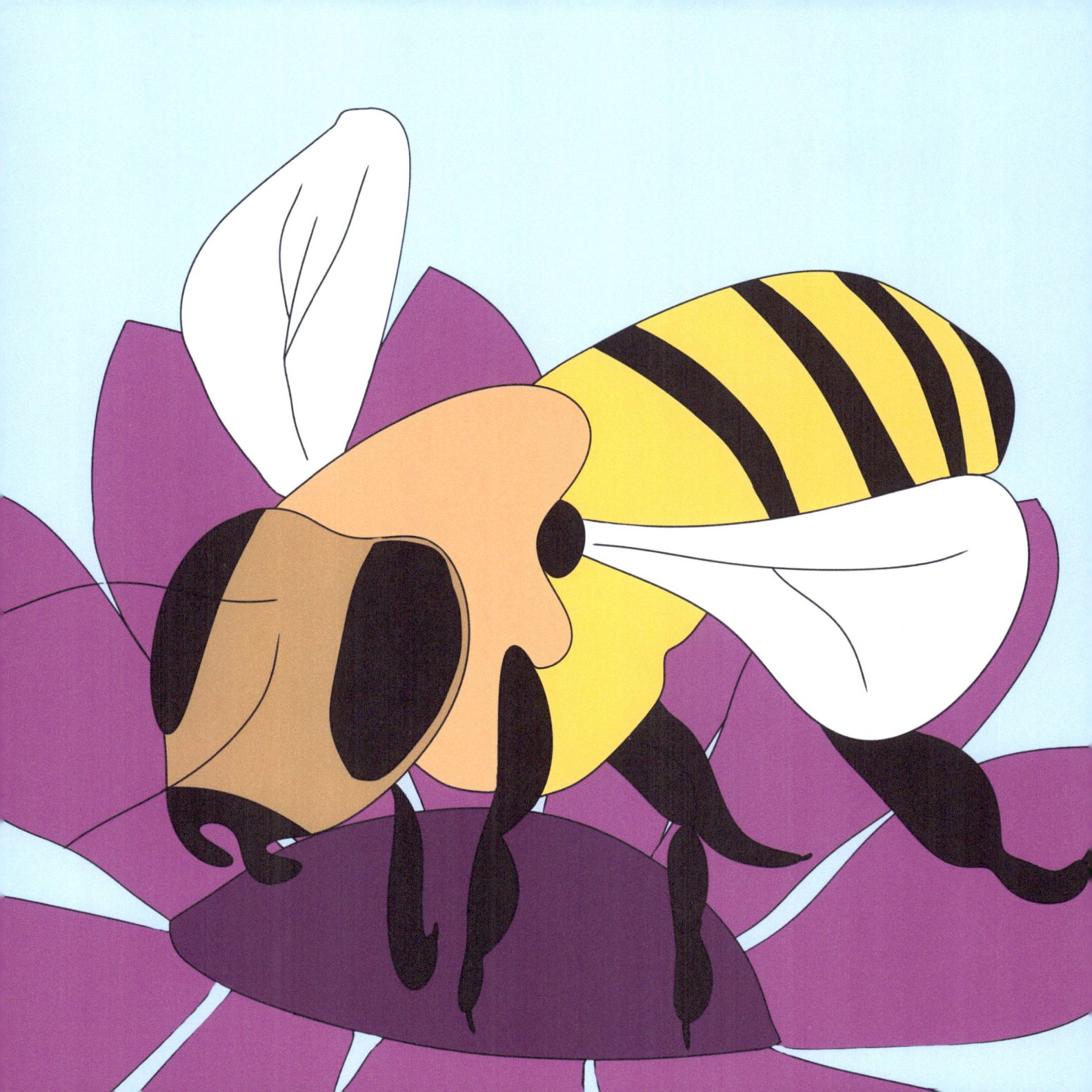

Milk for their babies

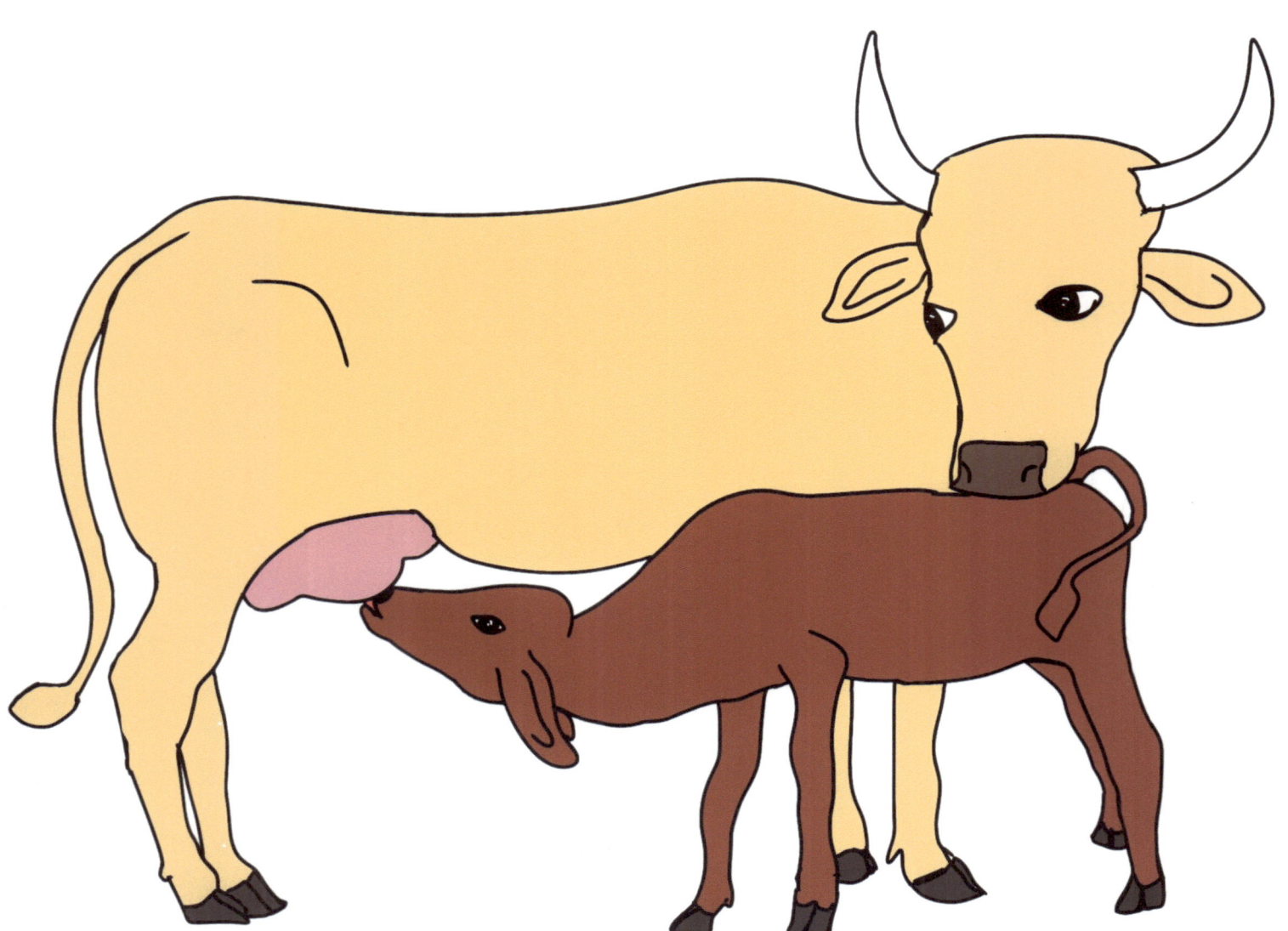

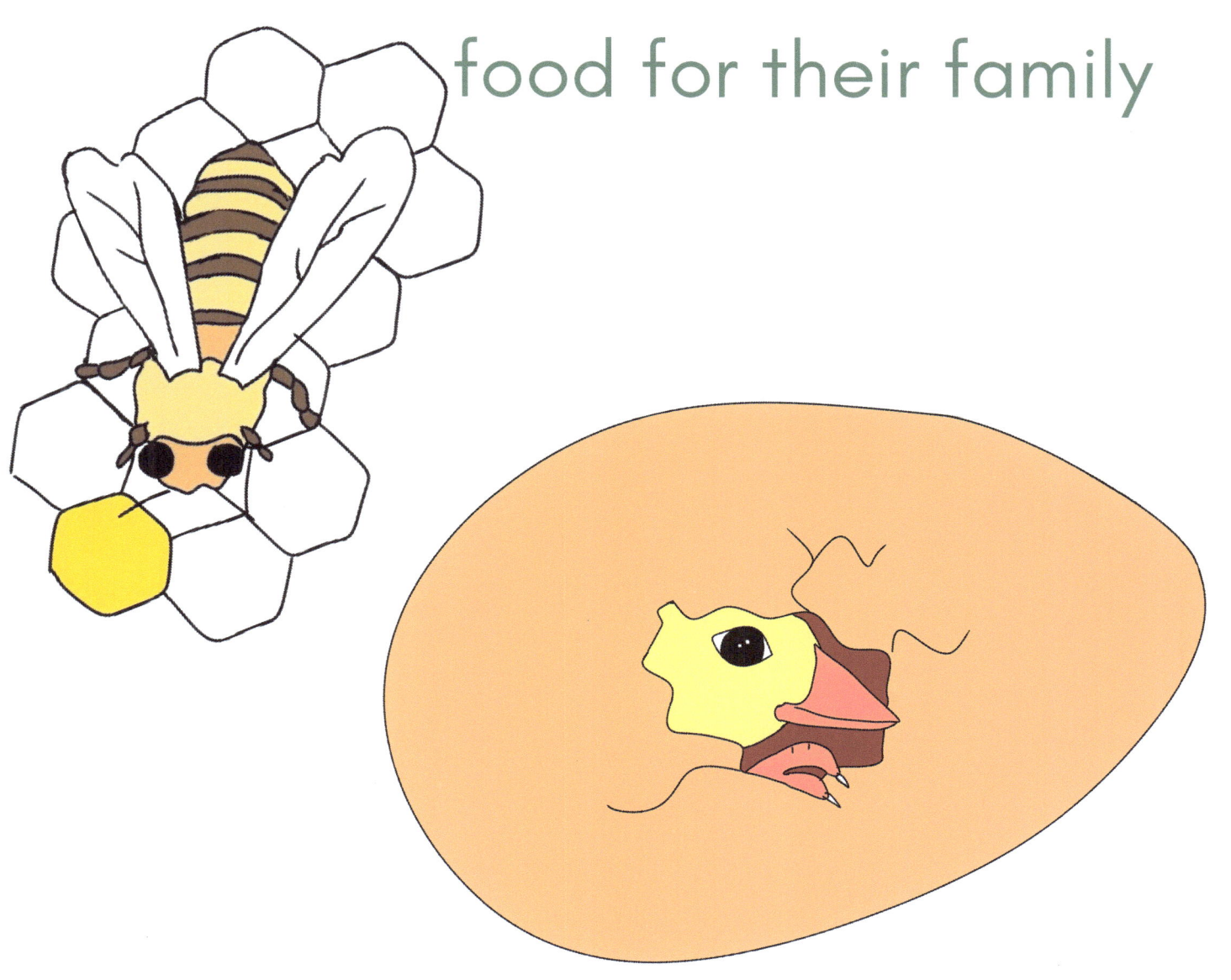

food for their family

eggs for new babies

For people to eat things made by animals, they take those things away and the animals get hurt.

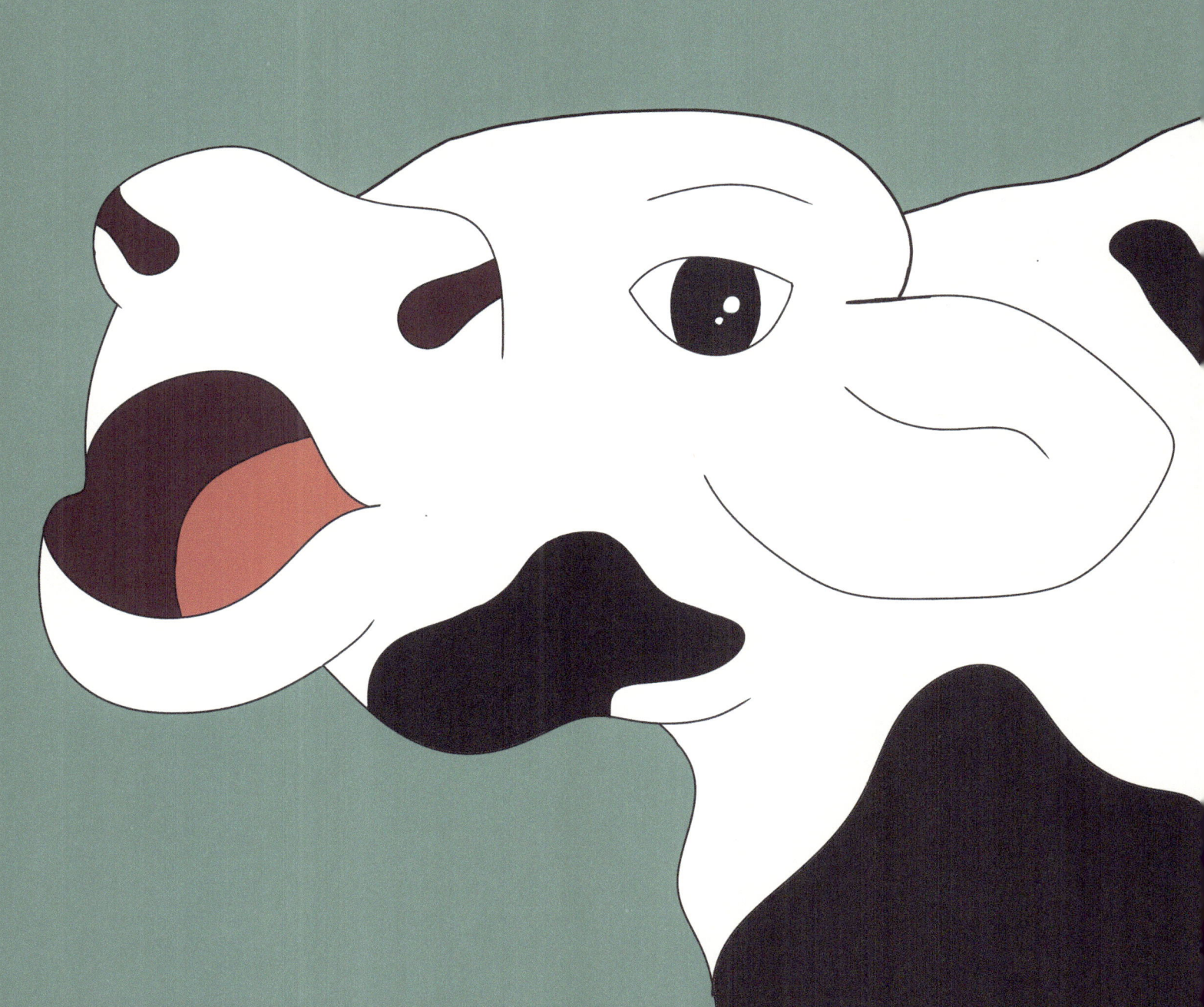

Our bodies can get all they need from plants

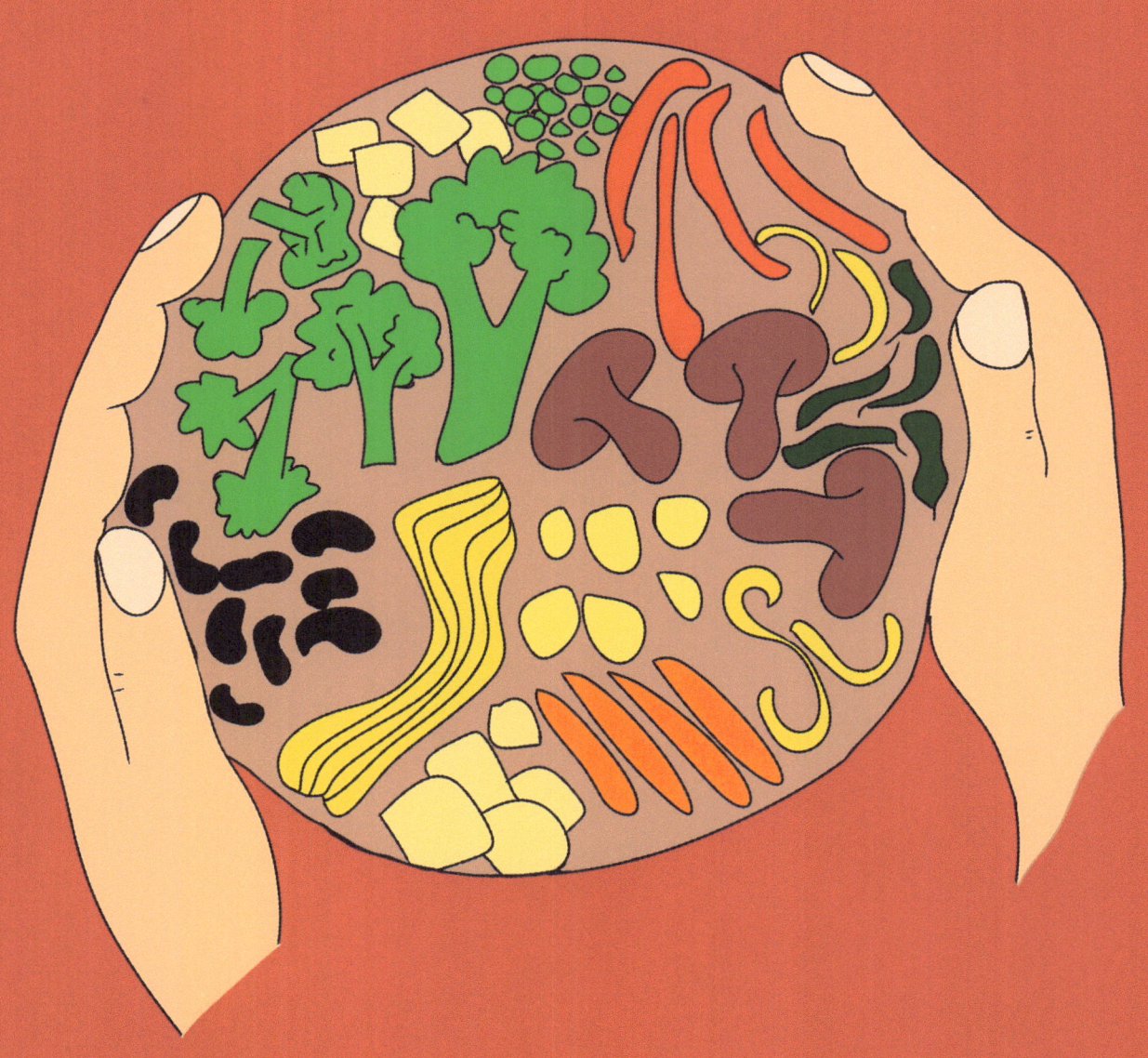

People who choose not to eat animals' bodies are called vegetarians

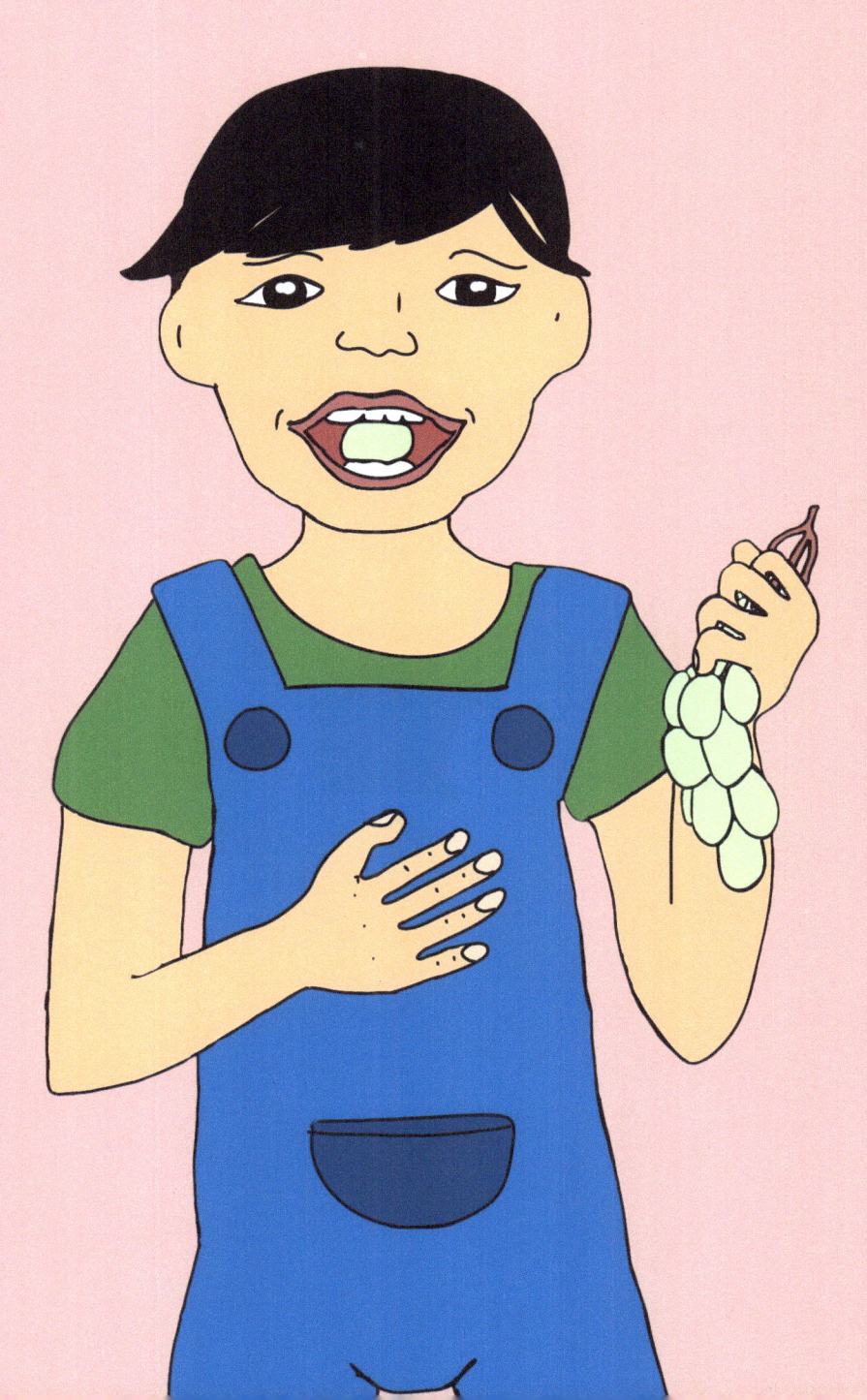

People who choose not to eat anything that comes from animals are called VEGANS.

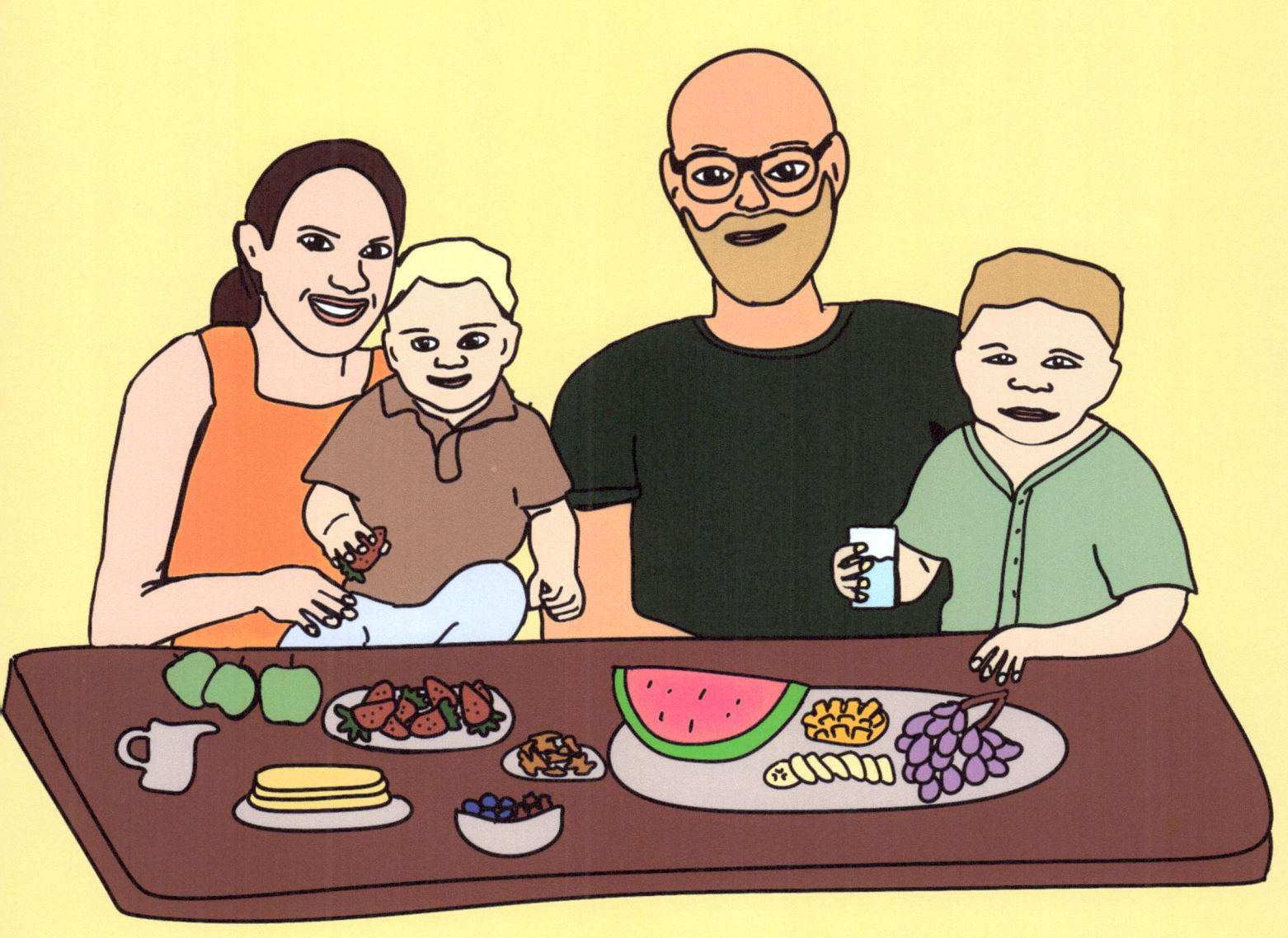

They only eat plants

We don't need to hurt
animals to nourish our bodies

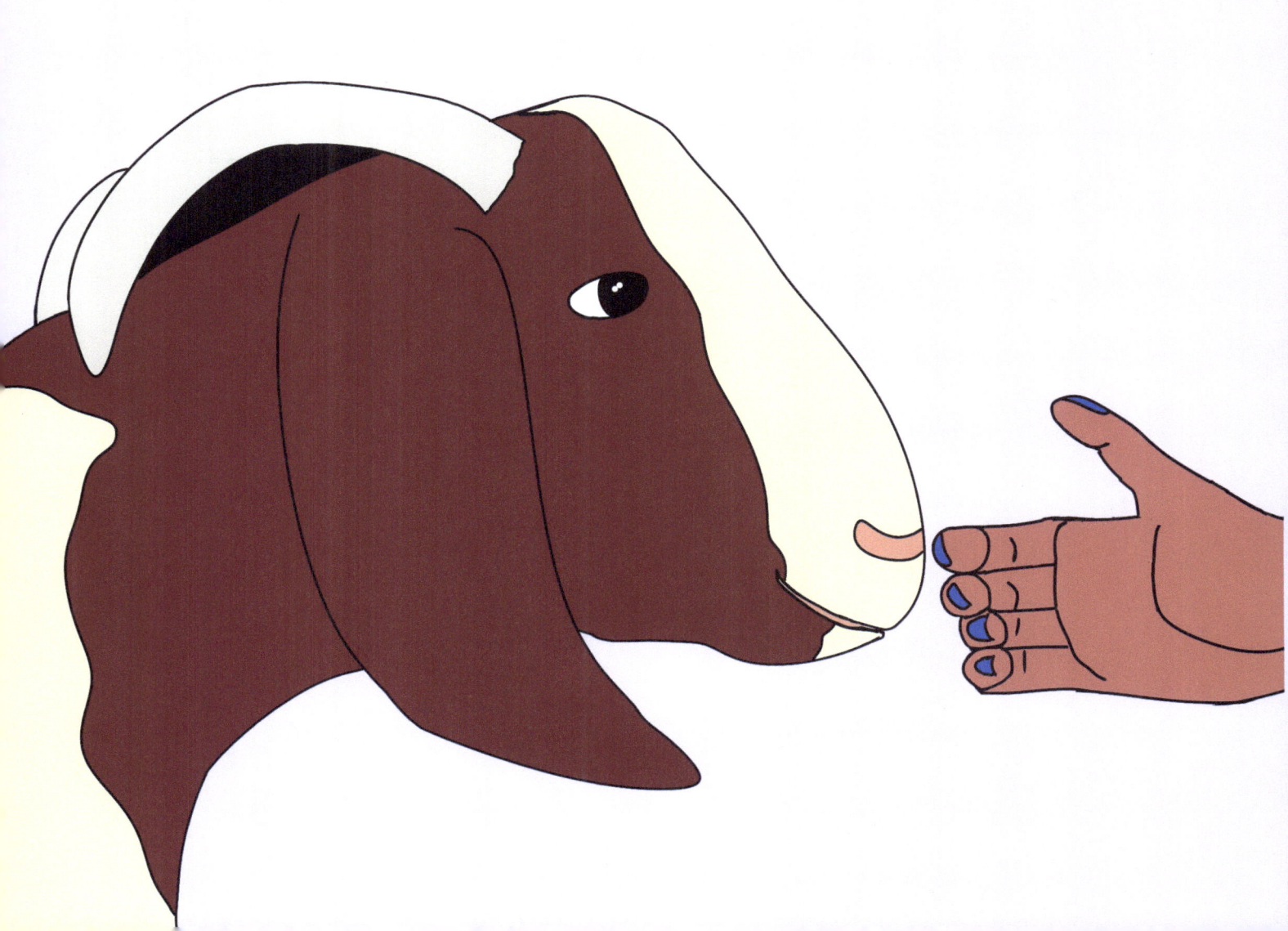

It's up to you to decide what to eat.

Be kind.

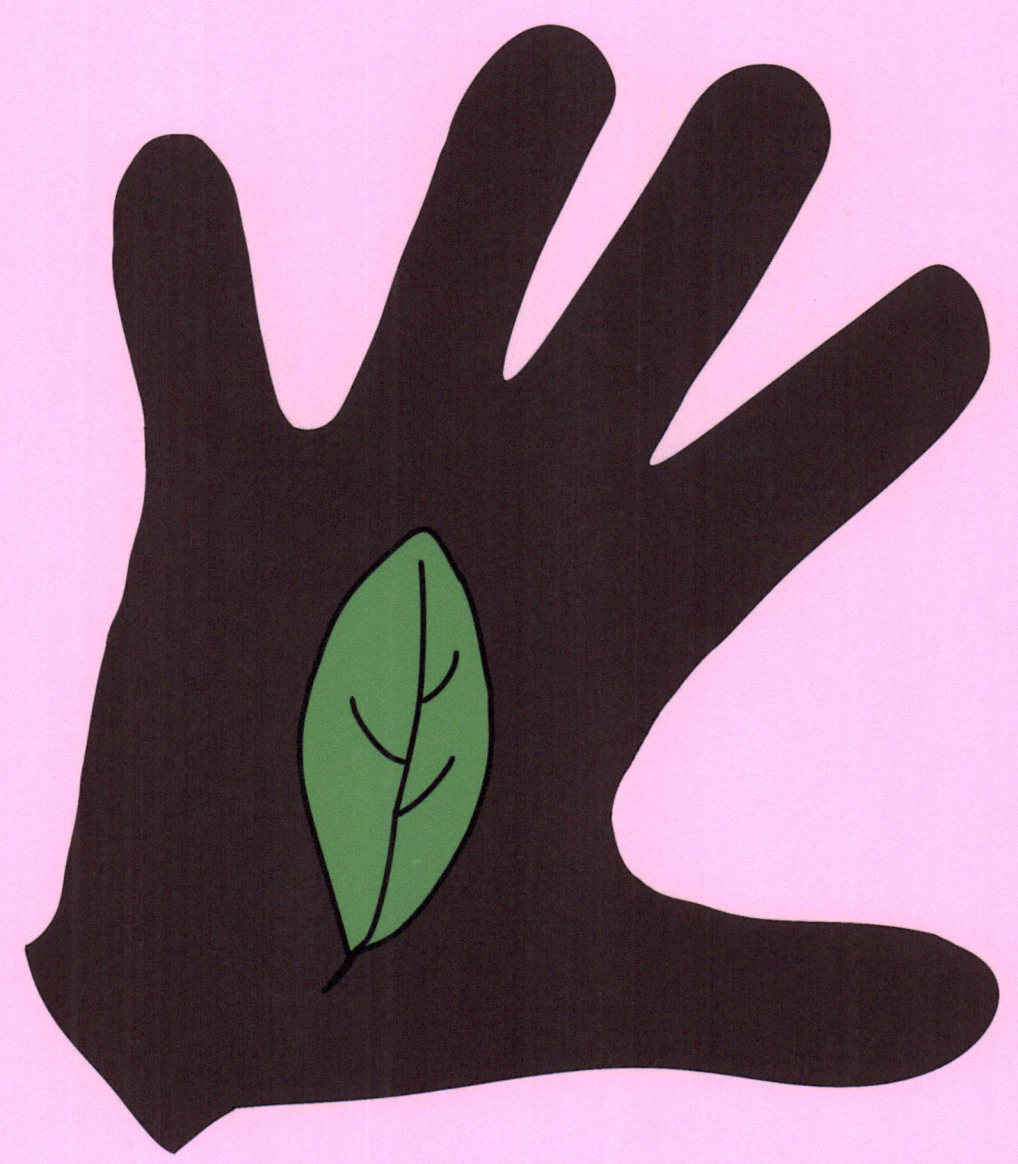

www.ingramcontent.com/pod-product-compliance
Lightning Source LLC
Chambersburg PA
CBHW041110070526
44583CB00003B/129